BEETROOT MIRACLES FOR WOMEN

A Closer Look at Gynecological Benefits

TABLEOF CONTENT

- Case studies or scientific studies highlighting hormonal improvements

Chapter 4: Beetroot and Menstrual Health

- The menstrual cycleand common menstrual issues

- Beetroot's potential effects on menstrual regularity

- Alleviating menstrual discomfort through beetroot consumption

- Personal stories of women experiencing improved menstrual health

Chapter 5: Beetroots for Fertility Enhancement

- Exploring factors affecting female fertility

- Beetroot's influenceon reproductive system function

- Nutrient components linked toenhanced fertility

- Real-lifeexperiences of women whoattribute improved fertility to beetroot

Chapter 6: Managing Menopause with Beetroot

- Understanding menopauseand its challenges

- Beetroot's role in mitigating menopausal symptoms

- Antioxidants and phytoestrogens in beetroot for menopause

- Testimonials from women finding relief through beetroot consumption

Chapter 7: Supporting Uterineand Ovarian Health

- Common uterineand ovarian health concerns

- Beetroot's potential effects on uterineand ovarian conditions

- Nutritional compounds and their impact on gynaecological health

- Medical expert insights on the useof beetroot as a complementary remedy

Chapter 8: Recipes for Gynaecological Wellness

- Nutrient-rich recipes featuring beetroot

- Smoothies, salads, soups, and other creative dishes

- Tips for incorporating beetroot into daily meals

- Balanced meal plans for women focusing on gynaecological health

Chapter 9: Beetroot and Holistic Wellness Practices

- Integrating beetroot intoa holistic health regimen

- Yoga, meditation, and stress reduction techniques

- The mind-body connection and its impact on gynaecological health

- Success stories of women who combined beetroot with holistic practices

Chapter 10: Safety, Precautions, and Consultation

- Important considerations before incorporating beetroot intoone's diet

- Potential interactions with medications or medical conditions

- Recommended beetroot consumption guidelines

- Encouragement to consult with healthcare professionals

Chapter 11: Conclusion: Embracing Beetroot for Gynaecological Wellness

- Recap of key points discussed in theeBook

- Encouragement for readers toexplore beetroot's potential benefits

- Empowerment to take chargeof gynaecological health through natural means

- Final thoughts and inspirational messages

INTRODUCTION

In the realm of women's health, gynaecological well-being stands as an integral pillar of overall vitality. The intricate danceof hormones, reproductive cycles, and bodily functions that women experience can be both empowering and challenging. As our understanding of holistic wellness continues toevolve, the roleof natural remedies has gained prominence. One such remedy that has captured attention for its potential to promote gynaecological health is the humble beetroot.

This eBook, "Beetroot Miracles for Women: A Closer Look at Gynaecological Benefits," embarks on a journey into the world of beetroot, exploring its remarkable nutritional profileand the potential it holds for supporting women's gynaecological wellness. From menstrual health and fertility enhancement to menopausal comfort and more, we will unravel the connection between beetroot and the various stages of a woman's reproductive journey.

Through evidence-based insights, real-lifeexperiences, and expert perspectives, this eBook aims toempower women with knowledge that can contribute to their well-being. As you delve into the pages that follow, you will uncover the multifaceted benefits that beetroot may offer, enriching your understanding of how nature's bounty can harmonize with the intricacies of the female body.

CHAPTER 1

UNDERSTANDING BEETROOT AND GYNAECOLOGICAL HEALTH

In theopening chapter of our exploration, we lay the foundation by delving into the world of beetroot and gynecological health. From its vibrant hue to its dense nutritional content, beetroot stands as more than just a kitchen staple—it's a potential ally for women's wellness.

Beetroot's Nutritional Powerhouse

We begin by unpacking the nutritional riches concealed within the beetroot. Bursting with vitamins, minerals, antioxidants, and dietary fiber, this unassuming root vegetableoffers a comprehensive spectrum of nourishment. Weexplore key nutrients such as folate, iron, and vitamin C, shedding light on how theseelements relate to gynaecological health. By understanding beetroot's nutritional composition, we lay the groundwork for its potential impact on various aspects of women's reproductiveand hormonal systems.

The Journey of Natural Remedies

As the world turns toward holistic approaches to health, the significanceof natural remedies becomes evident. We discuss the growing trend of seeking alternative solutions for gynaecological issues, offering insights into the synergy between traditional wisdom and modern science. This chapter highlights the importanceof considering natural remedies as complementary tools that work in tandem with medical interventions, fostering a balanced and integrativeapproach to well-being.

An Overview of theeBook

To navigate this journey comprehensively, we providea glimpseof the chapters that lieahead. From hormonal balanceand menstrual health to fertility enhancement and menopausal comfort, each subsequent chapter will dive deeper into the potential connections between beetroot and specific aspects of gynaecological wellness. As you read on, you'll uncover insights from scientific research, anecdotes from women who haveexperienced positiveoutcomes, and expert perspectives that shed light on the underlying mechanisms.

This chapter serves as a stepping stone, laying the groundwork for an informed exploration of the symbiotic relationship between beetroot and women's gynaecological health. As we venture forward, we invite you toembrace the possibilities that emerge when nature's bounty intersects with the intricate fabric of the female body.

CHAPTER 2

NUTRITIONAL POWERHOUSE: BEETROOT'S ESSENTIAL NUTRIENTS

In this chapter, we delve into the heart of beetroot's nutritional composition, uncovering thearray of essential nutrients that make it a potential gynaecological ally. From vitamins to minerals, antioxidants, and dietary fiber, weexplore how beetroot's rich profile can contribute to women's reproductive health and overall well-being.

The Many Faces of Beetroot

To truly understand the potential of beetroot in gynaecological health, we must first comprehend its nutritional complexity. We takea closer look at the vibrant colors and patterns present in beetroot, indicating the presenceof potent phytonutrients. These natural compounds are not only responsible for the root's vivid hues but also contribute to its potential health benefits.

Vitamins for Vitality

Weexplore the vitamins present in beetroot, focusing on key players such as vitamin C, vitamin B6, and folate. These vitamins are fundamental in supporting various aspects of gynaecological health, from immune function and hormonal balance to fertility and overall well-being. Through scientific insights, we delve into how each vitamin plays a role in women's reproductive systems.

Minerals that Matter

Minerals are the building blocks of bodily functions, and beetroot offers an array of them, including iron, potassium, and magnesium. Iron, for instance, is crucial for maintaining healthy blood hemoglobin levels and preventing anemia—a common concern among women. Weexplore the significanceof each mineral in promoting gynaecological health and delve into their potential impacts on menstrual cycles, fertility, and more.

Antioxidant Arsenal

At the coreof beetroot's health benefits lie its antioxidants, which combat oxidative stress and inflammation. We delve into the roleof antioxidants like betalains, betacyanins, and betanins in protecting cellular health, supporting immune function, and potentially reducing the risk of gynaecological conditions. By understanding theantioxidant-rich natureof beetroot, readers gain insight into its potential protectiveeffects on reproductiveorgans.

Fiber and Digestive Harmony

Dietary fiber, abundant in beetroot, plays a critical role in digestive health. Weexamine how fiber contributes to gut health, aiding in theelimination of toxins and supporting a balanced gut microbiome. A healthy gut is closely linked tooverall well-being, including hormone regulation and immune function, making dietary fiber an essential component of women's gynaecological health.

Nutrition and Gynaecological Wellness

In the closing sections of this chapter, we weave together the nutritional elements of beetroot and their potential impacts on gynaecological wellness. By understanding how vitamins, minerals, antioxidants, and fiber work in synergy, readers can grasp the multifaceted natureof beetroot's contribution to reproductive health.

Through a blend of scientific insights, real-world anecdotes, and expert perspectives, this chapter lays the groundwork for the subsequent exploration of beetroot's potential benefits in specific gynaecological aspects. As we journey forward, the connection between these nutrients and women's well-being becomes increasingly clear, illustrating the intricate interplay between nature's provisions and the complexities of the female body.

CHAPTER 3

BEETROOTS AND HORMONAL BALANCE

Within the intricate danceof a woman's body, hormones wield immense influenceover various aspects of health and well-being. In this chapter, we delve into the fascinating connection between beetroot and hormonal balance, exploring how the nutrients and compounds found in beetroot may play a role in supporting women's hormonal harmony.

Hormones: Orchestrators of Health

We start by delving into the world of hormones, explaining their pivotal role in regulating bodily functions, including menstrual cycles, fertility, and mood. Readers gain an understanding of the delicately balanced hormonal symphony that shapes women's experiences and the potential repercussions when this balance is disrupted.

Beetroot's Phytonutrient Arsenal

The vibrant hues of beetroot are not merely for aesthetic appeal; they signify the presenceof phytonutrients. We focus on phytonutrients like betalains, which exhibit antioxidant and anti-inflammatory properties. These compounds may contribute to hormonal balance by aiding in the detoxification processes that help eliminateexcess hormones from the body.

Regulating Insulin Sensitivity

Insulin sensitivity is crucial for maintaining hormonal balance, particularly in relation to conditions like polycystic ovary syndrome (PCOS) and diabetes. Weexplore how beetroot's nitrates can impact blood sugar regulation and insulin sensitivity. By addressing these factors, beetroot consumption may contribute to mitigating hormonal imbalances associated with insulin resistance.

Supporting Thyroid Health

The thyroid gland plays a central role in hormonal harmony, affecting metabolism, energy levels, and mood. We delve into the potential impact of beetroot's iodine content on thyroid function. While not a high sourceof iodine, beetroot can still bea valuable component of a balanced diet that supports thyroid health.

The Roleof Betaine

Betaine, another compound found in beetroot, has garnered attention for its potential to support methylation—a biochemical process that affects geneexpression and hormone regulation. Weexplore how betaine may contribute to hormonal balanceand geneexpression, shedding light on its potential mechanisms of action.

Harnessing Nature's Potential

In the concluding sections of the chapter, we draw together the threads of beetroot's potential impact on hormonal balance. By understanding the various ways in which beetroot's nutrients and compounds interact with the body's hormonal systems, readers gain insights into how this unassuming root vegetable may contribute to women's gynaecological wellness.

<h1 style="text-align:center">CHAPTER 4</h1>

BEETROOT AND MENSTRUAL HEALTH

The menstrual cycle is a cornerstoneof women's reproductive health, and its regularity and comfort contribute tooverall well-being. Thus weembark on an exploration of how beetroot might positively influence menstrual health, offering potential relief from discomfort and promoting a smoother cycle.

Understanding the Menstrual Cycle

We begin by revisiting the intricacies of the menstrual cycle, shedding light on its phases, hormonal fluctuations, and the rangeof experiences women may encounter. By understanding the menstrual cycleas a holistic process, readers can better grasp the potential intersections between beetroot and its various aspects.

Beetroot's Potential in Alleviating Menstrual Discomfort

Many women experience discomfort during menstruation, ranging from cramps and bloating to mood fluctuations. We delve into how theanti-inflammatory properties of beetroot's phytonutrients may offer relief from these symptoms. By reducing inflammation, beetroot has the potential toaddress the root causes of menstrual discomfort.

The Roleof Dietary Factors

Diet plays a crucial role in menstrual health, influencing hormone balanceand overall well-being. Weexplore how beetroot's nutritional components—such as iron, vitamins, and antioxidants—can contribute tooptimal menstrual function. Additionally, weexamine how dietary choices may impact estrogen levels and influence theoverall menstrual experience.

Nutrient Spotlight: Iron and Blood Health

Iron deficiency is a common concern among menstruating women, leading toanemiaand fatigue. Beetroot's iron content becomes a focal point as we discuss its role in supporting healthy blood hemoglobin levels. By addressing iron deficiency, beetroot may aid in maintaining vitality and reducing the risk of anemia-related symptoms.

Beyond the Monthly Cycle

In the closing sections of the chapter, we highlight the importanceof a holistic approach to menstrual health. This involves considering factors beyond dietary choices, such as stress management, exercise, and sleep. Beetroot's potential roleas a supportiveelement within a broader wellness strategy is underscored, encouraging readers to integrate it intoa balanced lifestyle.

CHAPTER 5

BEETROOTS FOR FERTILITY ENHANCEMENT

Fertility is a deeply personal and significant aspect of a woman's life, intertwining with her dreams of motherhood and family. In this chapter, we delve into the potential roleof beetroot in enhancing fertility, exploring how its nutritional profileand compounds might contribute to reproductive wellness.

Understanding Female Fertility

We begin by establishing a foundation of understanding around female fertility. From the intricate interplay of hormones to the conditions that can impact fertility, readers gain insights into the complex mechanisms that govern a woman's reproductive journey.

Beetroot's Nutritional Contributions

Central to beetroot's potential role in fertility enhancement is its robust nutritional composition. Weexplore how nutrients like folate, iron, and antioxidants in beetroot can support reproductive health. Folate, for instance, is vital for the development of a healthy fetus and can influence the conception process.

Antioxidants and Ovulatory Health

Theantioxidant-rich natureof beetroot is of particular interest when examining fertility enhancement. We delve into how antioxidants can combat oxidative stress, protecteggs,and optimizeovulatory function. By maintaining the health of eggs and promoting balanced ovulation, beetroot's antioxidants may contribute to improved fertility outcomes.

Nitric Oxideand Blood Flow

Nitric oxide, a compound found in beetroot, plays a crucial role in vasodilation—the widening of blood vessels. This effect can enhance blood flow to reproductiveorgans, potentially supporting a more receptiveenvironment for conception. Weexplore how beetroot's nitric oxide content may positively influence blood flow in the pelvic region.

Balancing Wellness for Fertility

In the closing sections, we underscore the importanceof a holistic approach to fertility enhancement. Weemphasize the roleof diet, exercise, stress management, and other lifestyle factors in supporting reproductive health. Beetroot, as a component of a well-rounded wellness strategy, may complement theseefforts by addressing specific nutritional needs.

By blending scientific insights with real-lifeexperiences, this chapter offers readers a comprehensive perspective that can inspire them to make informed choices as they navigate the path toward realizing their dreams of starting or expanding their families.

CHAPTER 6

MANAGING MENOPAUSE WITH BEETROOT

Menopause marks a significant transition in a woman's life, bringing with it a unique set of physical and emotional changes. In this chapter, we delve into the potential benefits of beetroot for managing menopausal symptoms and supporting women's comfort during this transformative phase.

Understanding the Menopausal Journey

We begin by exploring the intricacies of menopause, shedding light on the hormonal shifts and physiological changes that characterize this life stage. Readers gain insights into the challenges women may face, such as hot flashes, mood swings, and changes in bone health.

Beetroot's Potential in Alleviating Menopausal Symptoms

Theanti-inflammatory properties of beetroot's compounds becomea focal point as we delve into how they may offer relief from common menopausal symptoms. By reducing inflammation, beetroot has the potential to mitigate discomfort, regulate mood fluctuations, and support overall well-being.

The Roleof Phytoestrogens

Phytoestrogens, plant compounds with estrogen-like properties, are present in beetroot and can play a role in menopause. Weexplore how these compounds might interact with estrogen receptors in the body, potentially providing a mild estrogenic effect that can contribute to hormonal balance during menopause.

Bone Health and Nutrient Density

Menopause is associated with a decline in estrogen, which can impact bone health. Weexamine how beetroot's nutrients, including calcium, magnesium, and vitamin K, may contribute to maintaining strong and healthy bones. By supporting bone health, beetroot may mitigate the risk of osteoporosis—a common concern for women in later life stages.

Holistic Strategies for Menopausal Comfort

Readers areencouraged toexplore not only dietary changes but also mindfulness practices, stress reduction techniques, and other lifestyleadjustments that can contribute to menopausal comfort. Beetroot, as a part of this holistic toolkit, may offer multifaceted support.

As readers navigate through this chapter, they gain a deeper appreciation for the potential benefits that beetroot might offer in the context of menopause. By integrating scientific insights with personal narratives, this chapter equips readers with knowledge that can empower them toexplore natural approaches to managing menopausal symptoms, fostering a senseof control and well-being during this transformative life stage.

CHAPTER 7

SUPPORTING UTERINEAND OVARIAN HEALTH

The health of the uterus and ovaries is integral toa woman's reproductive well-being. In this chapter, weexplore the potential ways in which beetroot's nutritional components and compounds might contribute to the support and maintenanceof uterineand ovarian health.

Understanding Uterineand Ovarian Health

From the menstrual cycle to fertility and hormonal regulation, the uterus and ovaries play a vital role in a woman's reproductive system and have interconnected hubs of activity. Readers gain insights into the functions of theseorgans and the potential challenges they can face.

Beetroot's Nutritional Contributions

Central toour exploration is beetroot's nutritional profileand its relevance to uterineand ovarian health. Weexamine how nutrients like folate, vitamin C, and antioxidants can contribute to maintaining healthy tissues, supporting optimal hormone levels, and promoting overall well-being in these reproductiveareas.

Antioxidants and Cellular Protection

Theantioxidant-rich natureof beetroot becomes particularly significant when discussing uterineand ovarian health. Weexplore how antioxidants can protect cellular structures from oxidative stress, which can contribute to the prevention of cellular damageand the potential reduction of risks related to reproductive conditions.

Beetroot and Uterine Comfort

For many women, uterine discomfort is a recurring concern. Welook into the potential of beetroot's anti-inflammatory properties toalleviate symptoms such as cramping and bloating. By reducing inflammation in the uterine region, beetroot may providea natural approach toenhancing comfort during menstruation and beyond.

Balancing Wellness for Reproductive Health

Readers areencouraged to consider factors beyond nutrition, such as regular exercise, stress management, and hormonal balance. Beetroot, as a component of a holistic wellness strategy, may contribute to theseefforts by addressing specific nutritional needs.

CHAPTER 8

RECIPES FOR GYNAECOLOGICAL WELLNESS

In this chapter, we transition from theory to practice by providing a rangeof nourishing and delicious recipes that incorporate beetroot. These recipes are designed toempower women toeasily integrate beetroot into their daily meals, fostering gynecological wellness in a flavorful and enjoyable way.

Embracing Nutrient-Rich Cuisine

As weexplore the recipes that follow, readers gain insights into how various nutrients found in beetroot—such as vitamins, minerals, antioxidants, and dietary fiber—can contribute to specific aspects of reproductive well-being.

Beetroot in Smoothies

Beetroot-infused smoothies—havea versatileand convenient way toenjoy their benefits. Weoffer step-by-step instructions for crafting vibrant and nutritious smoothies that combine beetroot with other healthful ingredients like berries, leafy greens, and seeds. These recipes not only offer a burst of flavor but also serveas potential allies in hormonal balanceand menstrual health.

Salads Bursting with Flavor and Wellness

The next on our culinary exploration is beetroot-centered salads. We present a variety of salad recipes that showcase the harmony of colors, textures, and flavors. From mixed greens to feta cheese, nuts, and vinaigrette dressings, these salads providea delightful array of nutrients that can contribute tooverall gynecological wellness.

Soothing Beetroot Soups

Lastly is the realm of soups—a comforting and nourishing option. Our beetroot-based soup recipes offer not only warmth and flavor but alsoa potent blend of nutrients that can support menstrual health, hormonal balance, and more. From creamy concoctions to hearty broths, these soups providea canvas for women to indulge in the benefits of beetroot.

Balancing with Beetroot in Meals

Weemphasize that beetroot need not be confined to specific recipes but can be integrated into various meals. We provide guidanceon creative ways to incorporate beetroot into breakfasts, lunches, dinners, and snacks. From smoothie bowls to beetroot-infused pasta, these ideas inspire readers to think beyond traditional boundaries and explore new culinary horizons.

Balanced Meal Plans and Practical Tips

These meal plans showcase how beetroot can be seamlessly integrated intoa day's worth of meals, ensuring a consistent intakeof its potential benefits. Additionally, we share practical tips for meal preparation, storage, and sourcing high-quality ingredients.

By combining the richness of nutrition with the joy of cooking and eating, these recipes invite women to foster their gynecological wellness while savoring the pleasures of the table.

RECIPES FOR GYNAECOLOGICAL WELLNESS

We'll explore three categories of recipes: smoothies, salads, and soups. These recipes are designed to be nutritious, delicious, and easy to prepare, making it convenient for women toenjoy the benefits of beetroot.

Section 1: Beetroot Smoothies

Recipe 1: Berry-Beet Bliss Smoothie

Ingredients:

- 1 small beetroot, peeled and chopped

- 1 cup mixed berries (blueberries, strawberries, raspberries)

- 1 banana, peeled

- 1 cup spinach leaves

- 1 cup almond milk (or any preferred milk)

- 1 tablespoon chia seeds (optional)

- Honey or maple syrup to taste (optional)

Instructions:

1. Place the chopped beetroot, mixed berries, banana, spinach, almond milk, and chia seeds (if using) intoa blender.

2. Blend on high until smooth and creamy. If the consistency is too thick, add morealmond milk as needed.

3. Tasteand add honey or maple syrup if desired for added sweetness.

4. Pour into glasses and enjoy as a nutrient-packed breakfast or snack.

Section 2: Beetroot Salads

Recipe 2: Vibrant Beetroot Salad

Ingredients

- 2 medium beetroots, cooked, peeled, and cubed

- 2 cups mixed salad greens (lettuce, arugula, spinach)

- 1/2 cup crumbled feta cheese

- 1/4 cup chopped walnuts or almonds

- 1/4 cup dried cranberries

- Balsamic vinaigrette dressing

Instructions

1. In a large bowl, combine the cooked and cubed beetroot with the mixed salad greens.

2. Sprinkle crumbled feta cheese, chopped nuts, and dried cranberries over the salad.

3. Drizzle balsamic vinaigrette dressing over the salad just before serving.

4. Gently toss the ingredients to combineand coat with dressing.

5. Serve the beetroot salad as a refreshing and nutritious lunch or dinner option.

Section 3: Beetroot Soups

Recipe 3: Creamy Beetroot Soup

Ingredients

- 3 medium beetroots, peeled and diced

- 1 onion, chopped

- 2 cloves garlic, minced

- 2 cups vegetable broth

- 1 cup coconut milk (or heavy cream for a richer version)

- 2 tablespoons oliveoil

- Salt and pepper to taste

- Fresh dill for garnish

Instructions

1. In a large pot, heat theoliveoil over medium heat. Add chopped onion and minced garlic. Sauté until onions are translucent.

2. Add diced beetroot to the pot and cook for a few minutes, stirring occasionally.

3. Pour in the vegetable broth and bring toa simmer. Cover and cook until the beetroot is tender, about 15-20 minutes.

4. Usean immersion blender to puree the soup until smooth and creamy.

5. Stir in coconut milk or heavy cream toachieve the desired consistency.

6. Season with salt and pepper to taste. Adjust seasoning as needed.

7. Ladle the creamy beetroot soup into bowls, garnish with fresh dill, and serve warm.

Always encourageexperimentation and customization of recipes based on individual preferences and dietary restrictions.

CHAPTER 9

BEETROOT AND HOLISTIC WELLNESS PRACTICES

In this chapter, weexplore the intersection of beetroot's potential benefits with holistic wellness practices, showcasing how the mind-body connection can play a pivotal role in gynecological health. By integrating beetroot consumption with practices like yoga, meditation, and stress reduction, women can cultivatea comprehensiveapproach to well-being.

The Holistic Approach to Gynaecological Wellness

We begin by emphasizing the importanceof holistic wellness—nurturing not only the physical body but also the mind and spirit. By recognizing the interconnectedness of theseaspects, readers gain insights into how holistic practices can complement beetroot's potential benefits in fostering gynecological health.

The Mind-Body Connection

We delve into the profound connection between the mind and body, highlighting how stress, emotions, and thoughts can impact reproductive health. Readers gain a deeper understanding of how holistic practices like meditation, mindfulness, and yoga can influence hormone regulation, menstrual cycles, and overall well-being.

Beetroot and Stress Reduction

Stress is a pervasive factor that can influence hormonal balanceand gynaecological health. Weexplore how beetroot's nutritional components, such as antioxidants and nitrates, can contribute to reducing stress-related inflammation. Additionally, weexamine how theact of consuming beetroot mindfully can becomea form of stress relief in itself.

Yogaand Beetroot: Aligning Body and Mind

We delve into the practiceof yoga—an ancient discipline that unites physical postures, breath control, and meditation. We discuss how yoga can positively impact hormone regulation, alleviate menstrual discomfort, and promote stress reduction. By pairing yoga with the consumption of beetroot, women can synergistically enhance their gynecological wellness.

Meditation and Beetroot: Nurturing Inner Balance

The practiceof meditation is explored as a tool for cultivating inner harmony and emotional balance. We delve into how meditation's impact on the nervous system can indirectly influence hormonal balanceand reproductive health. Pairing meditation with beetroot consumption offers a holistic approach to nurturing gynaecological wellness.

Personal Journeys and Expert Insights

Throughout this chapter, personal stories from women who have combined beetroot consumption with holistic practices providea relatable dimension to the concepts discussed. Wealso include insights from experts in fields like nutrition, yoga, and mindfulness, offering guidanceon how these practices can be integrated into daily life.

Beetroot as a Holistic Companion

In the concluding sections, weemphasize that beetroot can serveas a supportiveally in one's holistic wellness journey. By pairing the nutritional benefits of beetroot with mindfulness practices, movement, and stress reduction, women can enhance their gynecological well-being from multipleangles.

By embracing practices that honor the mind-body connection, women can harness the power of synergy to cultivategynecological wellness that goes beyond the physical realm.

CHAPTER 10

THE FUTURE OF BEETROOT AND WOMEN'S GYNAECOLOGICAL HEALTH

As we look to the future, we contemplate how beetroot might continue to contribute to women's well-being and the broader context of natural remedies in modern medicine. Through emerging Research and Insights weexamineongoing studies, clinical trials, and emerging findings that shed light on the specific mechanisms by which beetroot's nutrients and compounds interact with the female reproductive system.

Collaboration between Scienceand Tradition

Weexplore theevolving relationship between scientific research and traditional wisdom when it comes to natural remedies. Scientific validation can enhanceour understanding of the potential benefits of beetroot while respecting the wisdom of traditional healing practices.

Beyond Beetroot: Integrating Holistic Approaches

While beetroot's potential benefits have been a focal point of this eBook, weexpand the perspective toencompass a broader array of natural remedies and holistic practices. We discuss how women can integrate various elements—such as dietary choices, herbal remedies, mindfulness practices, and medical interventions—in a way that supports gynecological health.

Personal Reflections: From Readers to Practitioners

Weencourage women to become proactive participants in their health journey, exploring new ways to integrate beetroot and other natural remedies into their lives. Additionally, we spotlight women who have transformed their passion for holistic wellness into careers, becoming practitioners, educators, or advocates for women's health.

Empowerment and the Path Forward

By acknowledging the potential benefits of beetroot and other natural remedies, women can take proactive steps toward enhancing their gynaecological wellness. We conclude by urging readers to continue their exploration and embrace the dynamic possibilities that the future holds.By reflecting on the insights shared throughout theeBook, they areequipped toapproach their gynaecological wellness with a senseof empowerment, curiosity, and open-mindedness.

The chapter serves as a fitting conclusion to theexploration of "Beetroot Miracles for Women," inviting readers toembracea future where the potential of nature's remedies intertwines with theevolving landscapeof women's health.

CONCLUSION

YOUR BEETROOT WELLNESS JOURNEY: PRACTICAL TIPS AND TAKEAWAYS

In this concluding chapter, we distill the knowledge, insights, and practical guidance provided throughout theeBook intoactionable takeaways. Weoffer readers a roadmap for embarking on their own beetroot wellness journey, empowering them to make informed choices that align with their unique needs, preferences, and goals.

Recapping the Journey

We begin by briefly summarizing the key themes, concepts, and chapters covered in theeBook. This recap serves as a reminder of the valuable insights gained and the holistic perspectiveon gynecological health that has been cultivated.

Crafting Your Beetroot Wellness Plan

Readers are guided through a step-by-step process of creating their personalized beetroot wellness plan. This plan encompasses dietary choices, lifestyleadjustments, and potential integration of holistic practices. We provide prompts and templates toassist readers in setting goals, defining strategies, and mapping out their wellness journey.

Setting Realistic Expectations

It's important to understand that holistic wellness is a gradual process that requires timeand patience. Weemphasize the significanceof setting realistic expectations and celebrating small victories along the way. By recognizing progress, readers can stay motivated and maintain a positiveoutlook.

Staying Connected and Informed

We highlight the valueof staying connected to theevolving landscapeof gynaecological health. Readers areencouraged to continue their exploration through books, onlineresources, and reputable health professionals. This ongoing engagement ensures that their understanding remains up-to-dateand well-rounded.

Harnessing the Power of Community

Creating a senseof community can bea powerful element of any wellness journey. We discuss the benefits of connecting with like-minded individuals who sharean interest in holistic health, gynecological wellness, and the potential benefits of beetroot.

Empowerment for a Lifetime

TheeBook concludes with a messageof empowerment. Readers areencouraged toembrace their roleas active participants in their health and well-being. By integrating the knowledgeand insights gained from theeBook, readers can continue to make informed choices that support their lifelong journey toward gynecological wellness.